The Magic of Natural Remedies

for Curing and Healing Naturally

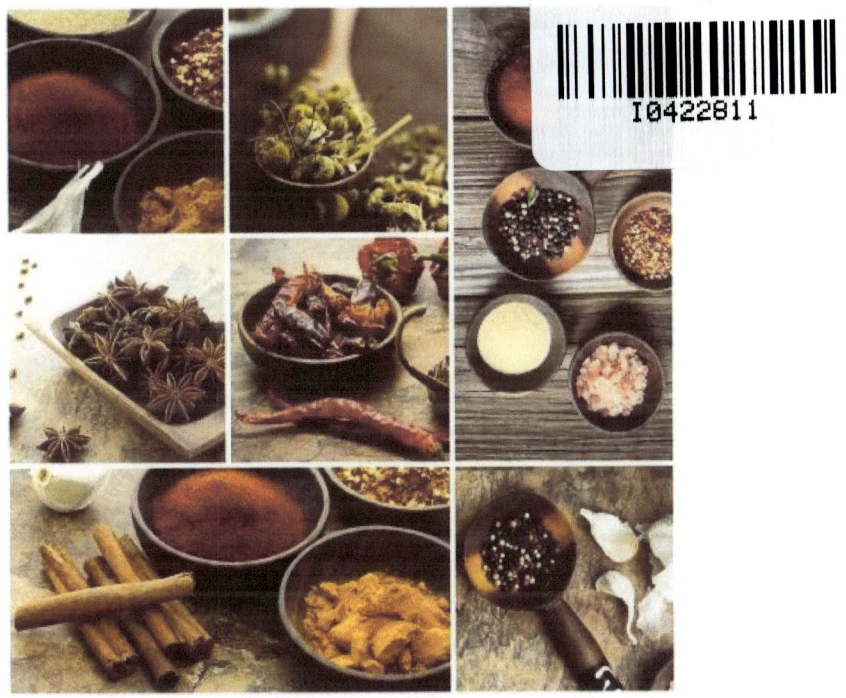

Dueep Jyot Singh
Health Learning Series
Mendon Cottage Books

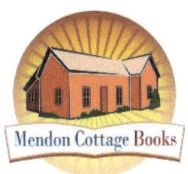

JD-Biz Publishing

Download Free Books!

http://MendonCottageBooks.com

Disclaimer

The information is this book is provided for informational purposes only. It is not intended to be used and medical advice or a substitute for proper medical treatment by a qualified health care provider. The information is believed to be accurate as presented based on research by the author.

The contents have not been evaluated by the U.S. Food and Drug Administration or any other Government or Health Organization and the contents in this book are not to be used to treat cure or prevent disease.

The author or publisher is not responsible for the use or safety of any diet, procedure or treatment mentioned in this book. The author or publisher is not responsible for errors or omissions that may exist.

Warning

The Book is for informational purposes only and before taking on any diet, treatment or medical procedure, it is recommended to consult with your primary health care provider.

Our books are available at

1. Amazon.com
2. Barnes and Noble
3. Itunes
4. Kobo
5. Smashwords
6. Google Play Books

Table of Contents

Introduction

If you are familiar with my magic series, you may have noticed that many of these books concentrate on just one magic herb or a magic spice, which is going to cure you. Naturally, the spices and herbs have been used since ancient times to help keep people healthy, beautiful, and also youthful.

Remember that not everybody in grandma's time or even in the time of our ancestors could afford to go to the doctor. In fact, physicians were only restricted to people who could pay their exorbitant fees. The rest of the common crowd made do with the knowledge that had been passed down to them, by their ancestors, and also from the knowledge gained through experimenting on their own.

This is how so many natural remedies came into vogue, and so many of them proved to be successful. Many of them were quack remedies, but this was because many of the ingredients which were used here were rather astonishing, when seen by a 21st century perspective. Nevertheless, there was some particular reason, why these quack remedies proved to be successful, because they had some material in them, which was able to cure people.

Now let us take for example, the use of goose grease, for rubbing on the scalp to make the hair grow faster. Goose grease is nothing but fatty oil. It moisturized the scalp. You could get the same results by rubbing in sheep fat.

So if our ancestors did not have one thing, they made do with something approximating that item, in their opinion. So one had to use goose grease and passed on this knowledge to his descendants, the coming generations began to believe that yes, this was the product, which would make your hair grow long, lustrous, and healthy. It would also keep your scalp dandruff free.

Now, what was the reason why so many people in ancient times kept healthy, even though they lived in unhygienic surroundings? Firstly, they had a strong constitution, and did not coddle themselves. They knew the value of the sun and the fresh air, and they stayed out as much as they could. They just came home to rest, eat, and possibly recuperate, if they suffered from some ailment or from injuries.

Also, they were very particular about their diet. They enjoyed plenty of fresh fruit and vegetables. They also drank fresh milk in large quantities whenever they could, as well as ate milk products like butter, butter, milk, cheese, and cottage cheese as often as they could, and when they could afford it.

The wealth of a tribe depended on that the amount of cows and goats they had. Other livestock was also very precious, but these came paramount. Whenever people of one tribe were attacked by people of other tribes, the cry went up "cows, pigs, horses, goats and sheep first, children second." The young children along with the animals were hidden away with the elders, who led the adults of the tribe do the fighting. This fighting was done, sometimes to the death, by the men and women of the tribe. The elders, who were unable to fight, were considered to be the people who would help the children survive, with knowledge about their ancient heritage.

This was the time when herbal lore was passed down to the generations from the elders of the tribe to the young next-generation and the youngest generation.

Now many of these herbal remedies, which I am going to tell you are made up of natural ingredients. I am going to try my best to make sure that they are easily available because my intention is to make sure that you get full benefits of all this ancient lore. Remember that all these remedies are time-tested. They may not have a scientific research stamp behind them, but they have come down through millenniums, and have proved their efficacy.

Time and time again, someone comes up with something new, and says that he has found that lanolin is amazingly good for skin, and he is going to use it in his special beauty treatments. His great-grandmother may just raise an eyebrow, and say, he is talking about sheep fat under a modern name!

So have fun browsing through this book, which is going to tell you all about the magic of natural remedies for curing your ailments naturally.

Am I talking about remedies, which have been in use in alternative medicine like Ayurveda, you may ask. Yes, some of these remedies are Ayurvedic, some of them are taken from other ancient medical, medicinal forms like Chinese, Greek, Egyptian, Persian and Mesopotamian, all of them ancient, all of them wise and all of them time tested and proven.

Let Us Start with

Keeping Our Teeth Healthy

The best natural foods to keep our teeth healthy are – buttermilk, honey, raisins, sesame, fenugreek, pomegranates, apples, carrots, sugarcane, dates, flour with the wheat bran included, lemons, mung, almonds, turmeric and radishes.

Foods to Avoid

If you are suffering from tooth trouble, make sure that you do not eat these products – yes, it is a long list, and you are going to be surprised to see how many of these items are conducive to tooth decay.

Cold drinks, tobacco, syrups, cokes, artificial juices with preservatives, ice cream, frozen foods alternating with hot foods, chocolates, white sugar, molasses, and even guavas are not very good for your teeth. Try reducing or removing them from your diet.

Remember to rinse out your mouth, after you have eaten something. I remember a child, complaining to his mom, who persisted on asking him to wash out his mouth, after he had lunch. Now this child had lunch at school, with his friends and he used to complain, "Mom,(*pronounced Mawwwww-hhhmmmm*) none of the other children do that. They laugh at me, when I go to the bathroom and wash out of my mouth."

Now peer pressure is definitely going to influence this child, and no child wants to be different from the others in his group. So his sensible mom thought up a really good alternative. She added an Apple to his lunch pack. She also told him to eat the apple after he had had his lunch. In this way she could be assured, that any item of food sticking to his teeth would be cleaned away, naturally and also, she was sure that her child would rather eat that apple, than getting himself laughed at by his other friends. Now this is wise psychology. This is what the ancients used.

Ginger Remedy

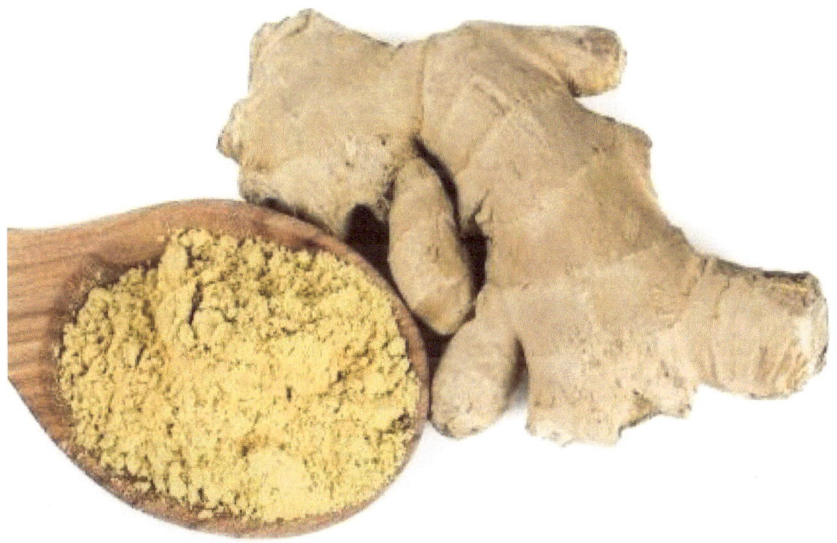

Get rid of toothache, if you do not have cloves around by taking a piece of raw ginger and putting it under the affected teeth. Then clench your mouth, so that you are biting on that piece of raw ginger. Allow the juice to collect any or mouth, and keep sucking on that ginger. You are going to see your tooth problem disappearing, thanks to this ginger juice. This is excellent, especially in the winter, when you suddenly find one of your teeth twinging, because of the cold. The ginger is going to keep you nice and warm!

Now this is one tooth ache remedy with which I saw a native wise man get rid of a toothache. It may look a little barbaric because it uses a toothpick to fill a partner in an aching and visible cavity.

Alum Turmeric Remedy

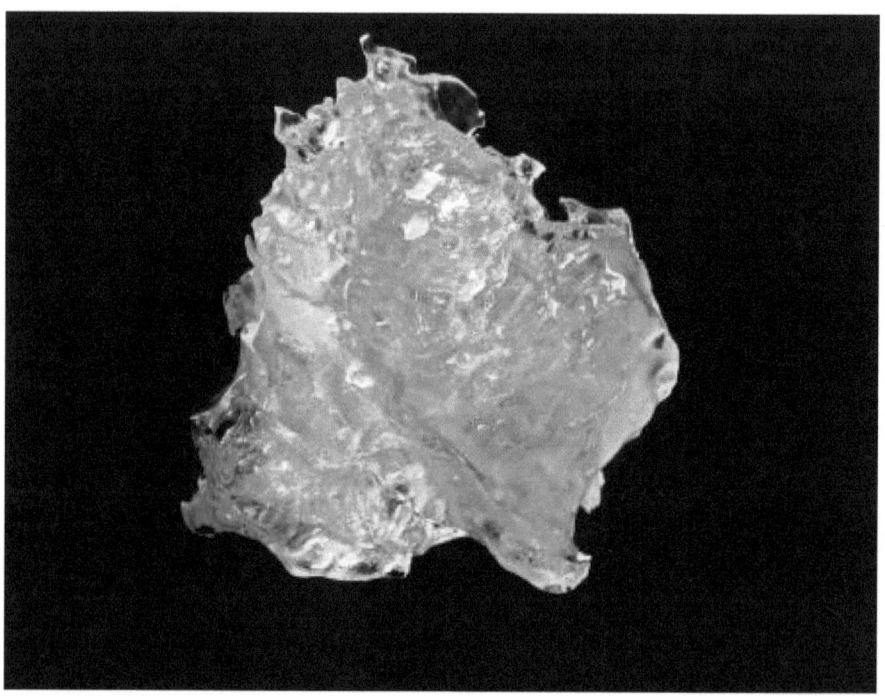

Take one teaspoonful of alum. Fry it on a griddle. This alum is going to swell up, when the water content in it dries. Powder it. Now take one fourth teaspoon powdered turmeric which you have roasted on the griddle. Mix both of them together. Now just take a toothpick, dip the end in this powder, and slowly and very carefully insert this powder into the cavity. The moment this medicine hits the aching nerves, you are going to find your tooth ache disappearing. However, you just need to do this once or twice at the most for really bad teeth, and that is that.

I saw it happening in front of my eyes. And as I was not brave enough to try this inserting a toothpick experiment on my teeth if they ever suffered from cavities, I went on the fact that prevention is better than cure binge.

I made sure that my teeth and gums are Healthy, by making up a mixture of this powdered alum and turmeric – hey, all of that powder was going to waste, but as he was a herbal doctor, he would use it. – and using it as a tooth powder with a little bit of salt added to keep my teeth glistening and healthy.

At least this is a much better way of keeping my teeth healthy, than the ancient Persians who used to brush their teeth with a powder of dried mutton bones. Well, here again, you can see the common sense. They got lots of calcium from those bones, as well as something abrasive, to get rid of any sticky deposit.

Turmeric tooth powder

Just dip your tooth brush in a little bit of turmeric, and brush all your teeth well. After you have done that, you can use your normal toothpaste. This turmeric is excellent to take care of your gums and possibly rotting teeth. I know about a person suffering from gingivitis, to whom the dentist had advised drugs to get rid of the swelling in the gums, before his teeth were extracted.

I told him all right, try this remedy, instead of taking those drugs. The swelling went down, and the infection got cured. And in 10 days. Astonishing. So make turmeric a part of your daily dental hygiene routine.

Turmeric tastes bitter, so you may not like its taste in the initial stages. People also think that this is going to stain your teeth. Do not allow the turmeric powder, when in wet condition to stain any of your clothes. If that happens, you will need to wash that affected area with lemon juice, and salt and put out in the sun so that the turmeric stain can bleach in the fresh air.

Colored Bottle Remedies

Glass green bottles work here, plastic bottles do not!

Now this is something, which I find very interesting. My mother is a very well-educated lady, but she definitely is not going to wear anything black on Monday. She also has her whole clothes cupboard coordinated according to the days of the week. Now, being an ex-science student and teacher myself, I was rather interested in her theory that particular days are given up to one particular color and you do not wear the color opposite to that color of the spectrum on that day.

So here is the secret for all of you.

Monday is the day for white, Tuesday for red, Wednesday for green, Thursday for yellow, Friday for Brown and Saturday for black and dark blue. Sundays are again for yellow and orange.

I do not know which ancient civilized nation began this theory about the planets ruling the days, but this color code is firmly entrenched in the minds of old people, coming down through the ages. And so my mother gets really worried, she sees me wearing black on a white day, and vice versa. Perhaps, it is autosuggestion, but things do not go well if that happens.

What a study of psychology. How you can affect your mind to behave in a way which makes you think that something went wrong, because it had to go wrong! I am not superstitious, touch wood, but I can understand how people got influenced with these ideas, told to them by their wise men and priests, who were the most powerful people in their society and tribe.

One of these ideas is drinking water, which has been kept overnight in a copper utensil. This is still very much in vogue in the East today. Well, this is the way in which you can prevent a copper deficiency in your body. The same thing goes for colored glass bottles.

Now, here we talk about a very important factor which helps in natural healing – the sun. Most of the natural medicines made in ancient times were sun cooked and sunbaked.

Skincare Remedy

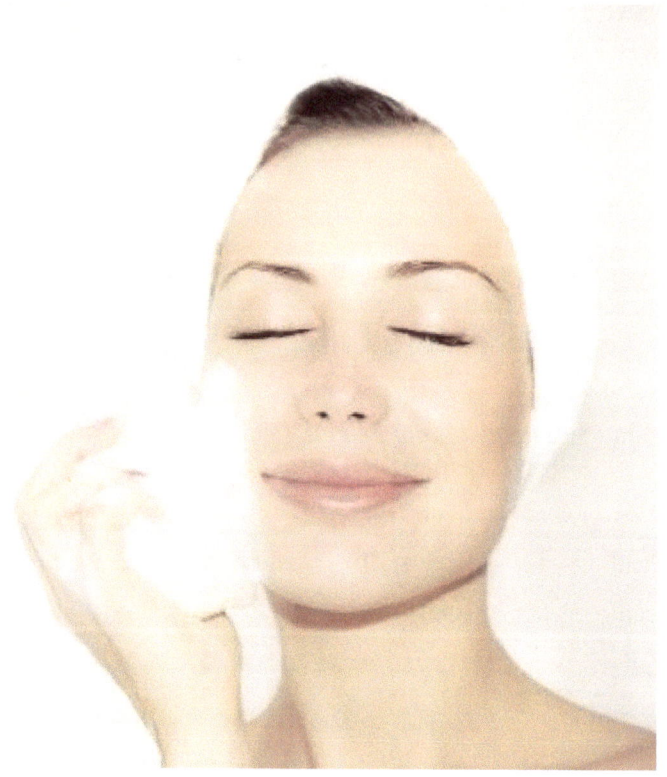

So get your green glass bottle ready. Your green plastic bottle is definitely not going to do its magic here. I have a range of assorted color bottles, borrowed from friends and relatives, who have just finished their whiskeys, brandies, and vodkas packaged in colored bottles. They suit me very well!

Take a green bottle and fill it up with coconut oil or your favorite moisturizing oil. Allow this bottle to cook in the sun for 20 days. Then apply the oil as a moisturizing lotion on your face and hands, and see all the blemishes disappear.

You can also moisturize your skin, by washing your face with one teaspoonful of yogurt in which you have put 2 teaspoons of honey. Wash your face after 10 minutes. You are going to find your skin texture and tone improving miraculously. This is also a good way in which you can get rid of chapped hands and feet.

Time-Tested Sore Throat Remedy

This remedy is for all those people who suffer from Streptococcus infections, in the throat. You find your throat swelling up, and there is pain in that area because of that, in connection. Try this remedy to take care of that sort throat.

Take one liter of water. Now put 2 tablespoons full of fenugreek seeds in it. Allow to boil on low heat for half an hour. This is going to reduce the volume of the water. Remove from heat, and wait till this is lukewarm. Now filter this decoction. Gargle with this warm decoction by filling your mouth with water and then gargling for 20 seconds before spitting out. Do this twice a day, or more often, depending on the seriousness of the throat infection.

This is an excellent remedy for tonsillitis. Also, if you find yourself suffering from phlegm and cough, this is an amazingly effective remedy.

I found one unexpected side effect, when I tried out this remedy to get rid of for tonsillitis infection last winter. My gums were rather sore, and I was worried whether they were infected. Gargling with fenugreek seeds cured my gums too, and any bleeding stopped because the gum infection had also been cured!

Sinus problems

Now this can be an embarrassment, especially when you are suffering from water dripping from your nose. Just take half a teaspoonful of ginger, and mix it in a cup full of water. Bring to a boil. [The more you boil the ginger, the more powerful it is going to be.] Then add half a teaspoonful of tea leaves, milk, and sugar, and prepare your normal cup of tea. Drink this before you are going to sleep. You are going to get cured within three days.

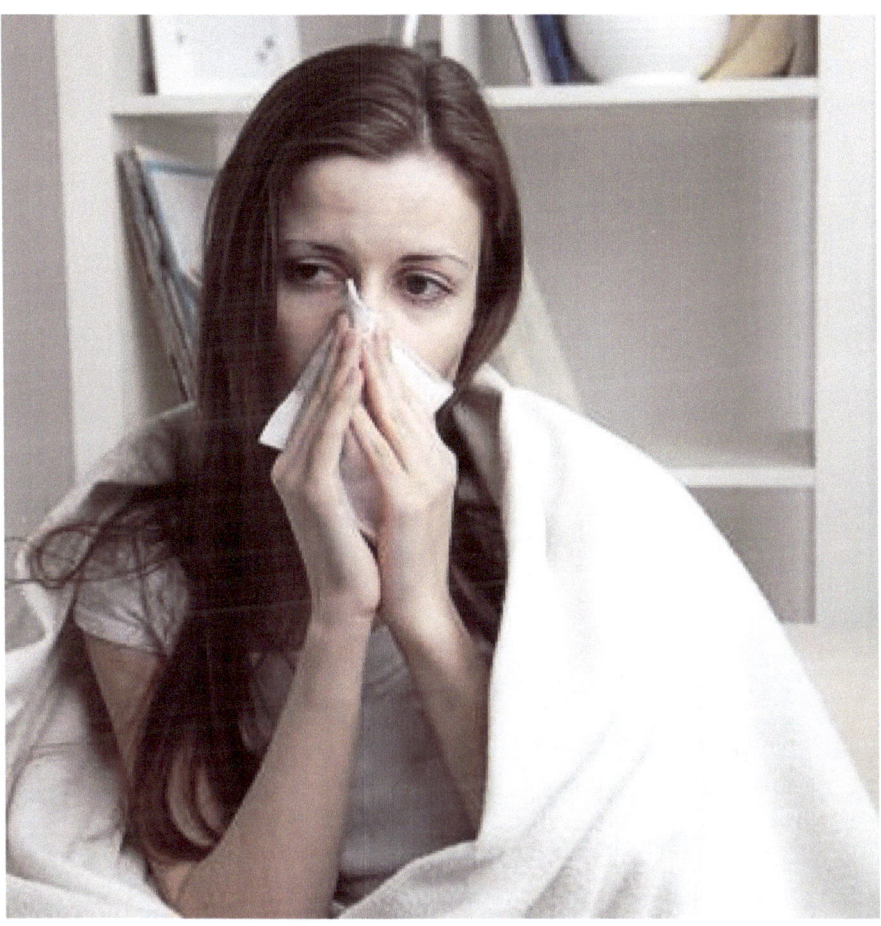

In the same way, if somebody is suffering from persistent cough, all he has to do is take a piece of ginger and keep chewing it. I remember giving the same remedy for people suffering from toothache. Hey, it is the ginger juice, which cures you.

Extremely Easy Cough Remedy

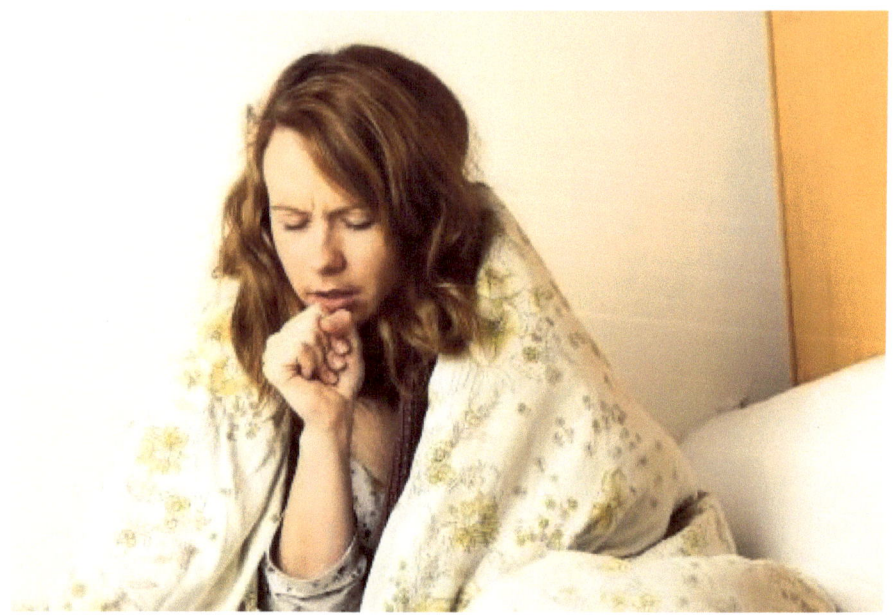

Now, you are going to wonder why I am giving you. So many remedies, for coughs and colds, but then, these are the ailments which trouble us the most. It is said that anybody who finds an effective remedy for a cold is going to be a millionaire. I have not found a time-tested immediate remedy for a cold yet, but I can give you one for coughs, persistent, chronic and phlegm coughs, and other cough related ailments.

Just take hundred grams of rock salt and keep it ready whenever you suffer from coughs. This is going to be the best investment you ever made. Because you just need to dip it once in water.

Original rock salt is pinkish in color. It was discovered in what is now Pakistan by Alexander the great's horses, more than 2000 years ago. It is marketed in powdered form in America under the name of Himalayan salt. There are other rock salt beds all over the world, so when you get a chunk, preserve it.

Rock Salt Remedy

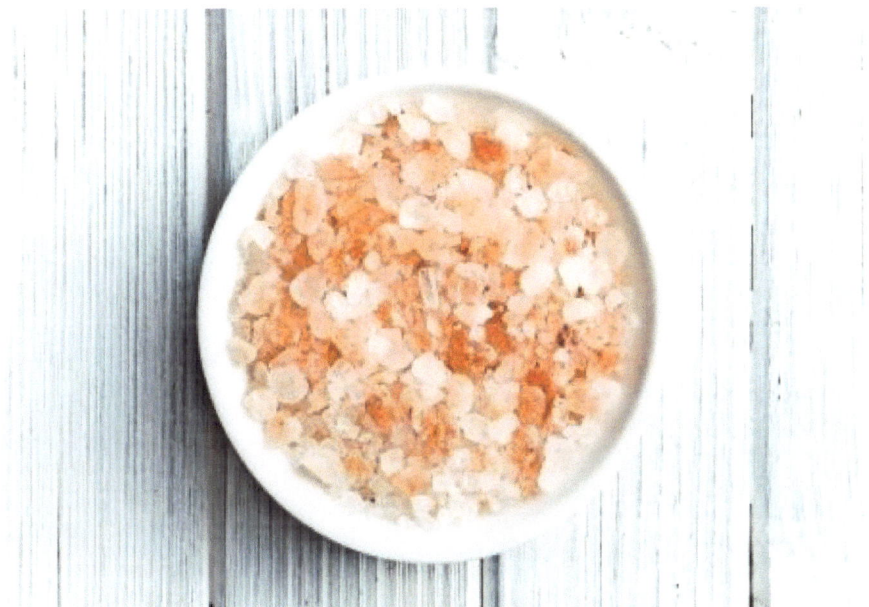

Just pick up this rock salt chunk with tongs and heat it on the griddle. When it starts to turn red-hot, dip this chunk into half a cup of water. Dip it just once, and pull it out. Then drink that water in just one huge swallow. This is what you are going to do before you go to sleep for the night. This drastic salty treatment every night for three days is going to cure your cough especially when it is a wet nasty cough.

You are going to let that chunk of salt dry in the air before you store it away again in your air tight container. In this manner, you can use it again and again.

Here is another way in which you can use this rock salt to cure your cough. Take 125 g of water, and add just half a teaspoon of rock salt. Allow to boil until the volume is half in quantity. Drink this morning and evening, and you are soon going to see your cough disappearing.

This remedy is not suitable for all those people suffering from high blood pressure.

For those people who cannot manage salt because of HBP, here is my next lifesaver.

Turmeric Remedy

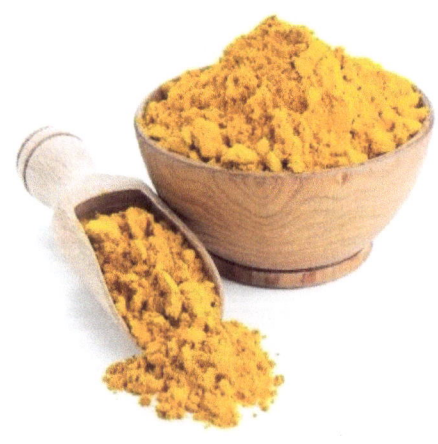

Take a small teaspoon of roasted and ground turmeric – remember that this is bitter in taste – and add it to half a teaspoonful of honey. Mix them in a little water and heat. Make the patient gulp this down when it is lukewarm and before he goes to sleep. Two days and he is going to see himself cured.

You can also take this in a form of one small teaspoon powdered turmeric, with a spoonful of sugar with a little bit of warm water swallowed after.

Banana remedy for asthma

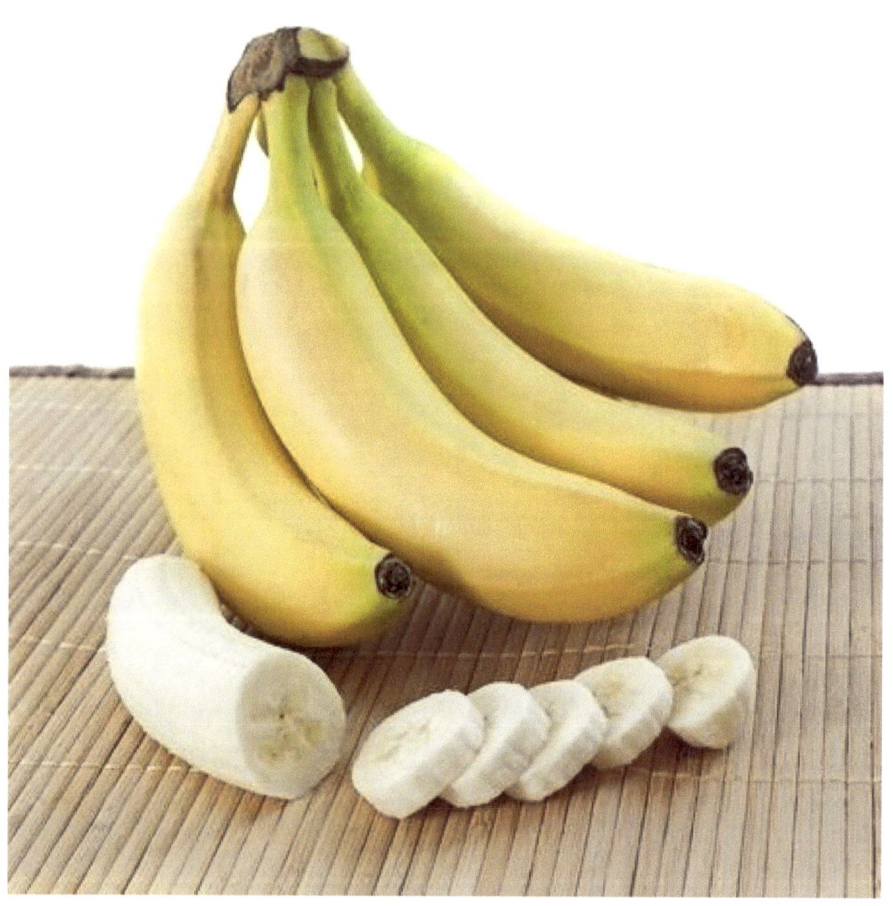

Now this is something extremely unusual, but I found an herbalist in one of the small towns curing people for miles around with his banana remedy.

Take a banana. **Do not peel it.** Make a longitudinal cut in it with a sharp knife. Now fill the cart with filtered powdered black pepper. Then, without peeling the banana, wrap the banana up in a banana leaf. Tie it up with some thread and allow the pepper to work its magic. Do this in the morning.

In the evening, take that still wrapped banana and roast it on the fire until the outer leafy covering is burned. When it is cool, peel the banana and eat the pepper fruit.

You will need to do this for 15 to 20 days. Then get back to me with happy sounds of success. And remember to pass on this remedy to all those people around you suffering from asthma problems.

Bananas are amazingly effective to cure asthma and breathing problems. You can also try this remedy, in which you are going to be using banana leaves yet once again.

Dry some banana leaves in the shade – the shady portion of your sunny porch – and burn them in a clay pot, your oven or in a utensil until you just have ashes. Then filter these ashes and put them in a glass bottle. There you are, you have your medicine ready.

How to use this medicine? Take half a teaspoonful of really old molasses, [the older the better,] and dissolve it in 2 tablespoons water. Now put ¼ teaspoons of this banana powder in this water, and allow to wait 10 minutes. You just need to take this once a day.

You will have to take this for about one to 1 ½ months in order to cure yourself.

Natural remedies for heart attack prevention

Our very hectic, as well as sedentary lifestyles have made us very prone to possible heart ailments, especially when we are not bothered about diets.

Here are two natural remedies which are going to help you a lot.

Mint Leaves Remedy

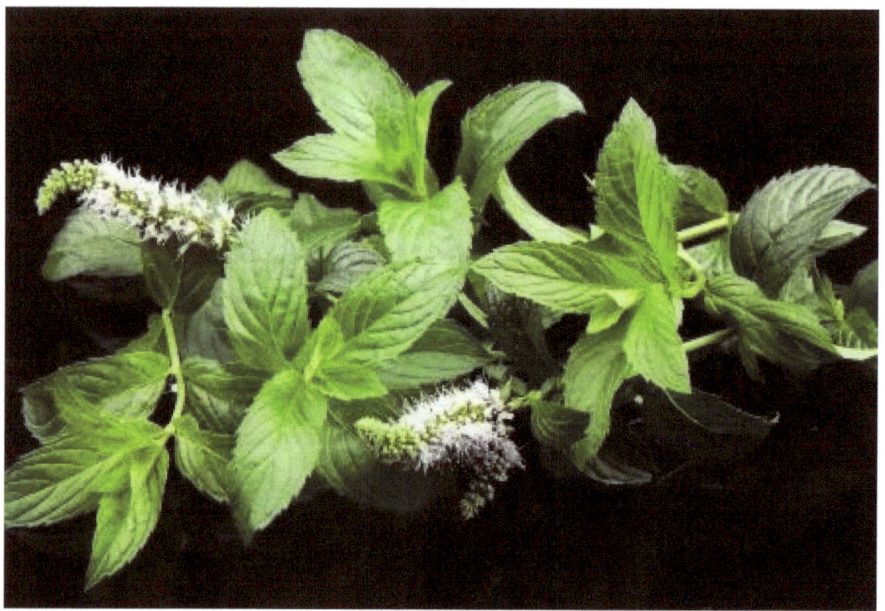

This is extremely easy, if you have mint leaves growing in your garden. Just dry a fistful of mint leaves in the shade. Filter them after you have powdered them. Morning and evening, you are going to take two pinches of powdered mint leaves, with one pinch of powdered pepper. Then take a swallow of water.

This is an excellent way to keep your stomach healthy, and also helps in preventing potential heart attacks. That is because of the pepper.

Bengal gram – black chickpea Remedy

Take 25 g of roasted black chickpeas **Cicer arietinum** made into a powder with a glass of water, or in a glass of milk or with yogurt, once every day. – 25 g is about 1 ½ tablespoons full.

This is considered to be a very efficient remedy, especially when you have already suffered from heart attack, and there is a chance of that occurring again. I would suggest that you grind about half a kilogram of these roasted chickpeas, and powder them. Place in an airtight container. Then you do not have to bother about roasting them and grinding them afresh every single day.

This is also considered to be very efficacious, if you are also suffering from diabetes.

Best Natural Diet for People Suffering from Heart Problems

If you are prone to heart problems, you definitely know all about foods to eat and which foods to avoid. Your doctor has told you all about them. You have read plenty of information about these foods on the Internet. I am just adding myself to the long line of advisors giving you some tips for your own good.

Stop eating fried items, rice, meat products, eggs, and also stopped drinking and smoking. Instead, start including these items to your diet – buttermilk, raisins, black Bengal gram soaked at night and eaten in the morning, fenugreek seeds, apples, garlic, pomegranates, Indian gooseberry, and papaya.

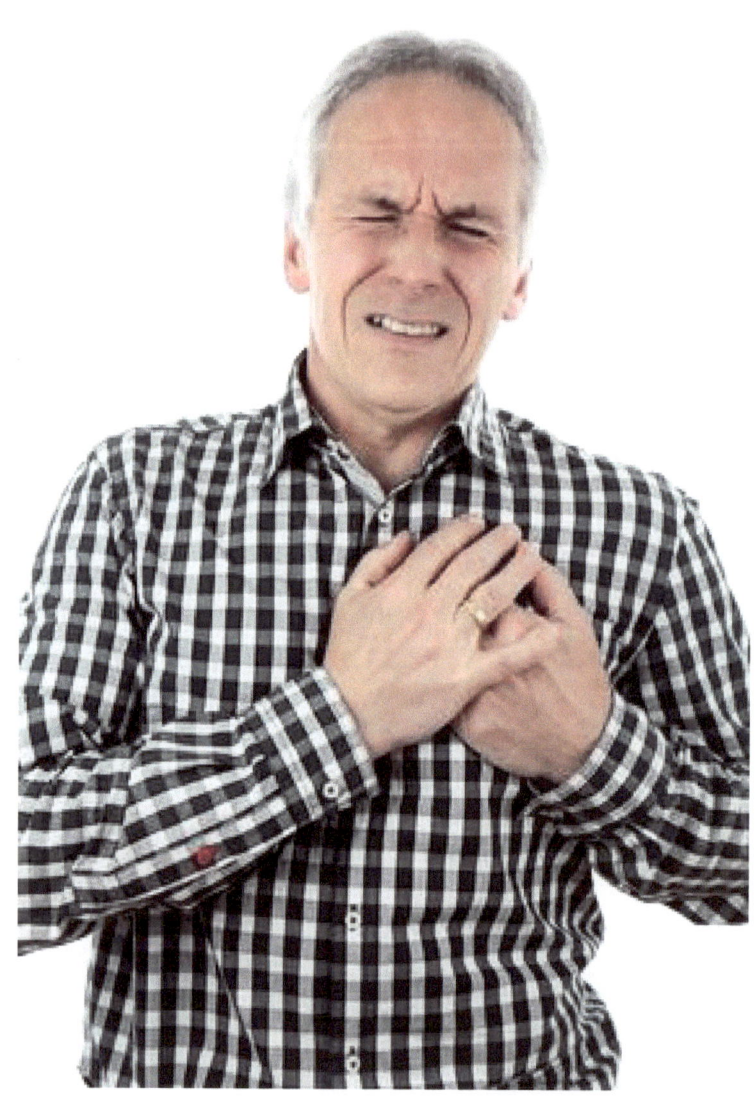

Tonic to Strengthen Your Heart

Try out this remedy to help heal your heart. It consists of 10 g of raisins and 10 g of rock candy – you may try Honey, if you are not a diabetic patient – boiled in 250 g milk. Drink this for breakfast, every morning. 15 days and you are so going to find an improvement, especially if you find your pulse rate quite high.

Lowering Cholesterol

Raisins Remedy

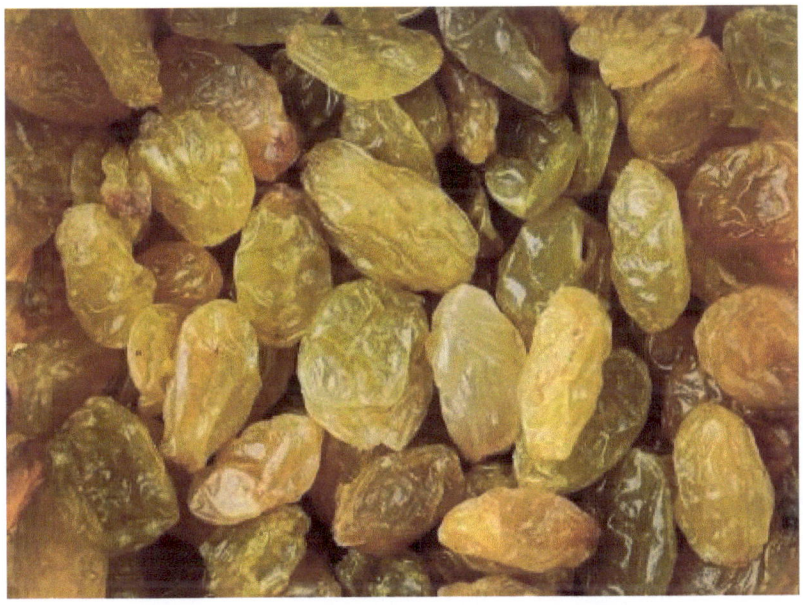

Raisins have been in use since ancient times to keep you really healthy and fit. You can lower your cholesterol by soaking six raisins and 24 – 30 chickpeas in half a cup of water overnight. Then early next morning, chew them up well and also drink the water. This is going to keep you healthy, especially when you use this remedy in the summer.

This remedy is not good for those people suffering from diabetes.

Garlic for Lowering Cholesterol

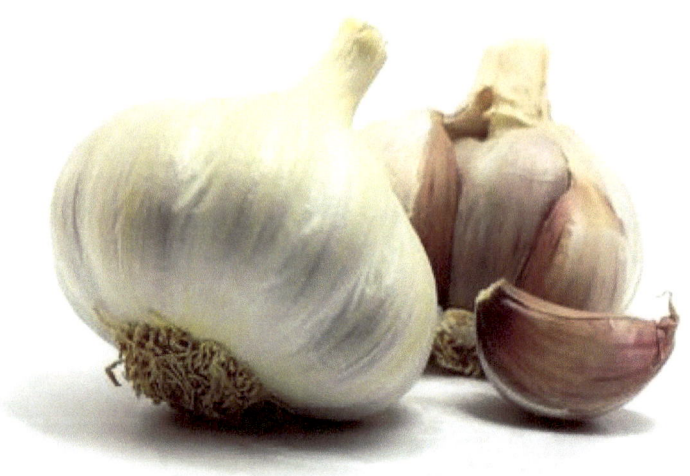

This is something I remember as a child seeing my father doing, every night before going to sleep. He used to take one clove of garlic, peel it and eat it raw. But then he was trying to prevent cholesterol from occurring! Never mind, he kept his system infection free.

For people suffering from cholesterol and who want to get rid of it, you need to take 2 fat cloves of garlic, peel and chop them. Then you have to eat them **first thing in the morning on an empty stomach, with a little bit of water.** Of course, the breakfast you eat afterwards, before running for the office is going to remove all that garlicky smell. But this is an extremely effective way to lower cholesterol. I know of a person, who suffered from high cholesterol – 325 or so. One month of this treatment and it came down to 220. Another month more and it lowered even further to 140.

With more than 250 scientists all over the world, proving again and again that garlic is excellent for heart health, and spending their time in researching something which has already been proved by other scientists, even I can say that the sulfur in the garlic helps in high blood pressure. Someone said the same thing millenniums ago.

Remember **not** to eat garlic in the summer.

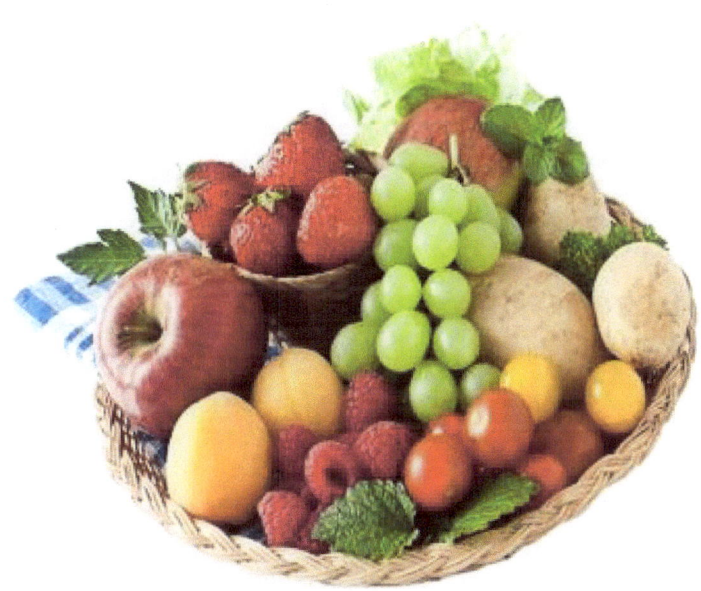

Summer-y Healthy Food Does Not Include Garlic in that particular season.

Here are some precautions, which I would advise when you are doing a garlic remedy.

Do not eat sour stuff. Also, do not eat spices, pickles, molasses and a high-protein diet, including meat and eggs. That is because the garlic is going to produce enough of heat in your body in order to cure you, so more foods which are hot in nature like meat is only going to aggravate your condition.

Instead, eat more milk products. Try vegetarian food. Do not exercise too much.

If you find that eating garlic makes you feel warm, stop eating it for a couple of days till your system gets back into normal. Instead, start increasing milk and milk product items in your diet.

Who Should Avoid Garlic

People suffering from urinary problems, bile problems, piles and even ladies expecting should keep away from garlic. If you happen to be very thin and anorexic with eating disorders, garlic is definitely not for you.

No wonder anorexic French, Spanish and Italian models eating something with garlic in it, find themselves losing their temper ever so often. One is because of this continuous dieting, when your body demands food and you are not giving it the proper necessary nutrition. The other is eating hot garlic.

People living in hot tropical zones, especially in the summer should not eat garlic.

Garlic for Gout

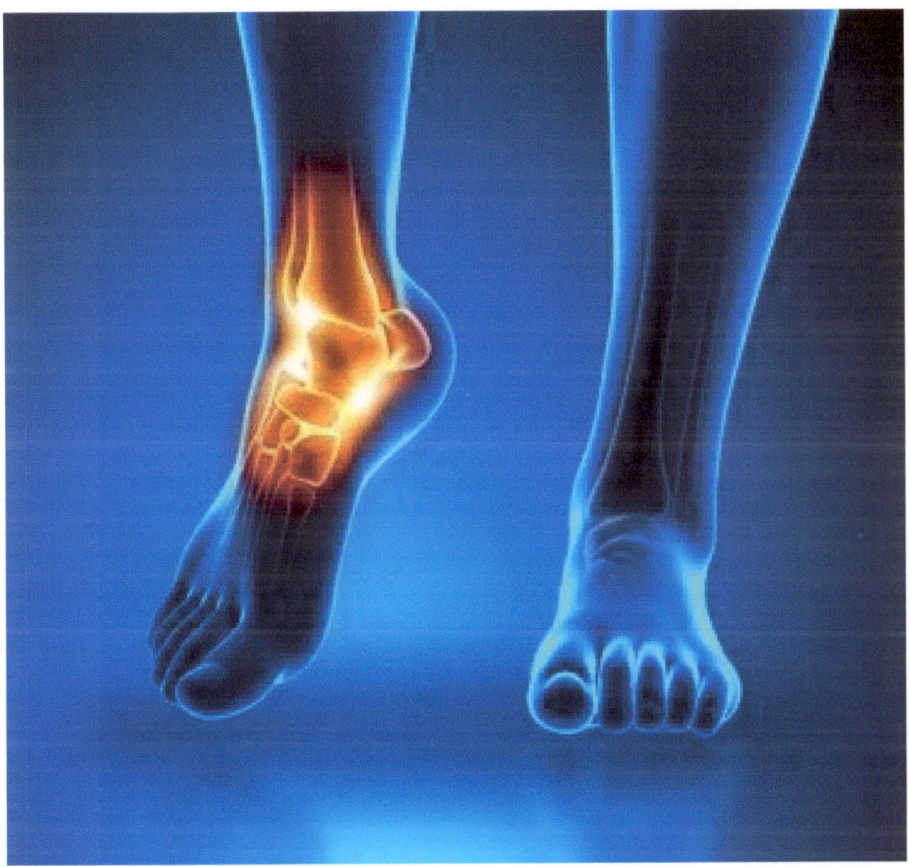

This remedy is for all those people suffering from gout – whether chronic or a recent development. Take five cloves of garlic. Chop them up into small pieces, after you have peeled them and boil them in half a liter of milk. Now this very effective garlic milk has been in use for millenniums to help cure go out. Filter it and remove the garlic. Drink this for six weeks every night before going to sleep.

Many of us are definitely not milk drinkers, because we are not very certain whether we are getting the real thing or we are getting soya bean milk.

Do not eat anything sour while continuing this treatment. Also, rich and fatty as well as fried foods should be avoided. Eat easy to digest foods. Try adding more fruit and vegetables to your diet in order to get rid of the toxic wastes causing gout.

Garlic to Cure Sciatica

This Remedy is going to cure your sciatica problems within the month. Eat four cloves of garlic, first thing every morning, just like you are swallowing down capsules. Along with that, you are going to have a chutney for lunch, which is going to be made up of four capsules of raw garlic, salt, chilies, and turmeric. Take 1 teaspoon of this chutney with your lunch. You are going to find you cured in a month. If the problem is severe, you can continue for another month, but the answer is – no sciatica , ever again.

Sweet Almond Oil

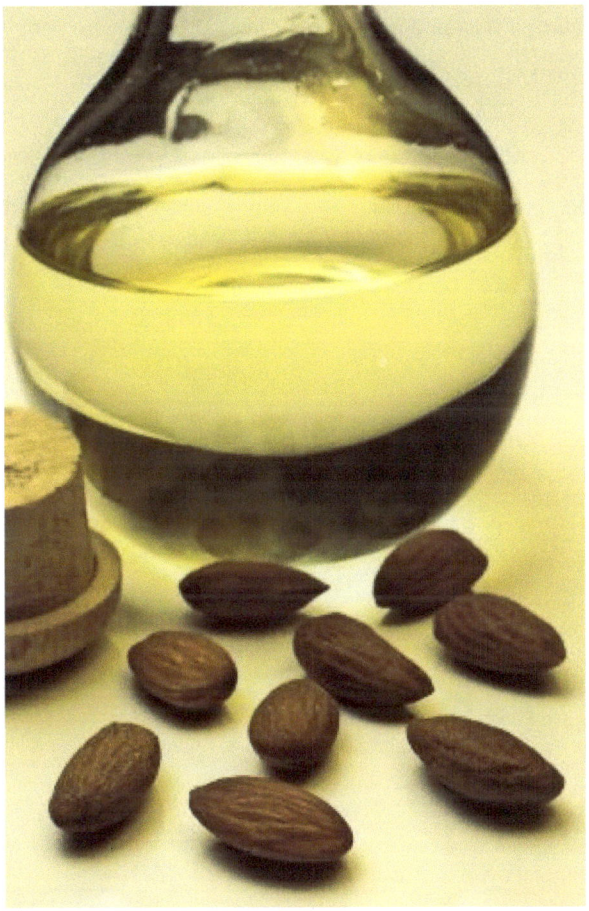

Sweet almond oil is rather expensive because it is so much in demand as a skin moisturizer and beautifier. But in these, it has been used as a natural remedy for curing constipation. People put two drops of sweet almond oil in the glassful of milk they drink for breakfast. No worries about tummy problems or constipation ever.

Now this was a remedy told to me by a person suffering from high blood pressure, as well as continuous headaches. He just dripped five drops of sweet or just ordinary almond oil, both work equally effectively into his nostrils. And then he took a deep snort, so that he inhaled that oil. He does this every night without fail before going to sleep.

Not only did this help cure his headaches, but he says that it has improved his high blood pressure. No harm in trying it out. Come to think of it, let me try it from tonight, to see if it gets rid of my headaches caused by sinus!

Conclusion

This book introduces you to just a fraction of the amazing time-tested remedies out there, which you can use to cure yourself. Why does it take so long for these remedies to work, you may ask. All you have is to go to the nearest doctor, and ask for a dose of quick acting medicine. You are going to get cured really fast and that is what your top priority is, is not it?

Well, natural medicine does not work that way. It intends to cure the ailment from the root, without any harmful side effects. You may find yourself suffering from harmful side effects by taking chemical drugs. And then you are going to go back to your doctor again and ask him for medicines to get rid of those side effects, brought on about by taking medicines in the first place. This is going to be a complete and totally vicious circle.

This does not happen when you are taking natural remedies. That is because the medicines that you are taking have been in use for millenniums, and are made up of totally natural products. All the elements of nature have been put to use to give you the best results. Naturally, these natural products are going to look at the root of the illness and try to cure it.

So here are some remedies, which I am sure you are going to find useful. Look out for more magic remedies books where you are going to get information about the wisdom of the ages.

Live Long and Prosper!

Author Bio

Dueep Jyot Singh is a Management and IT Professional who managed to gather Postgraduate qualifications in Management and English and Degrees in Science, French and Education while pursuing different enjoyable career options like being an hospital administrator, IT,SEO and HRD Database Manager/ trainer, movie scriptwriter, theatre artiste and public speaker, lecturer in French, Marketing and Advertising, ex-Editor of Hearts On Fire (now known as Solstice) Books Missouri USA, advice columnist and cartoonist, publisher and Aviation School trainer, ex- moderator on Medico.in, banker, student councilor ,travelogue writer … among other things! One fine morning, she decided that she had enough of killing herself by Degrees and went back to her first love -- writing. It's more enjoyable! She already has 48 published academic and 14 fiction- in- different- genre books under her belt.

When she is not designing websites or making Graphic design illustrations for clients , she is browsing through old bookshops hunting for treasures, of which she has an enviable collection – including R.L. Stevenson, O.Henry, Dornford Yates, Maurice Walsh, C.N.Williamson, Sapper, Bartimeus and the crown of her collection- Dickens "The Old Curiosity Shop," and so on… Just call her "Renaissance Woman" - collecting herbal remedies, acting like Universal Helping Hand/Agony Aunt, or escaping to her dear mountains for a bit of exploring, collecting herbs and plants, and trekking.

Check out some of the other JD-Biz Publishing books

Health Learning Series

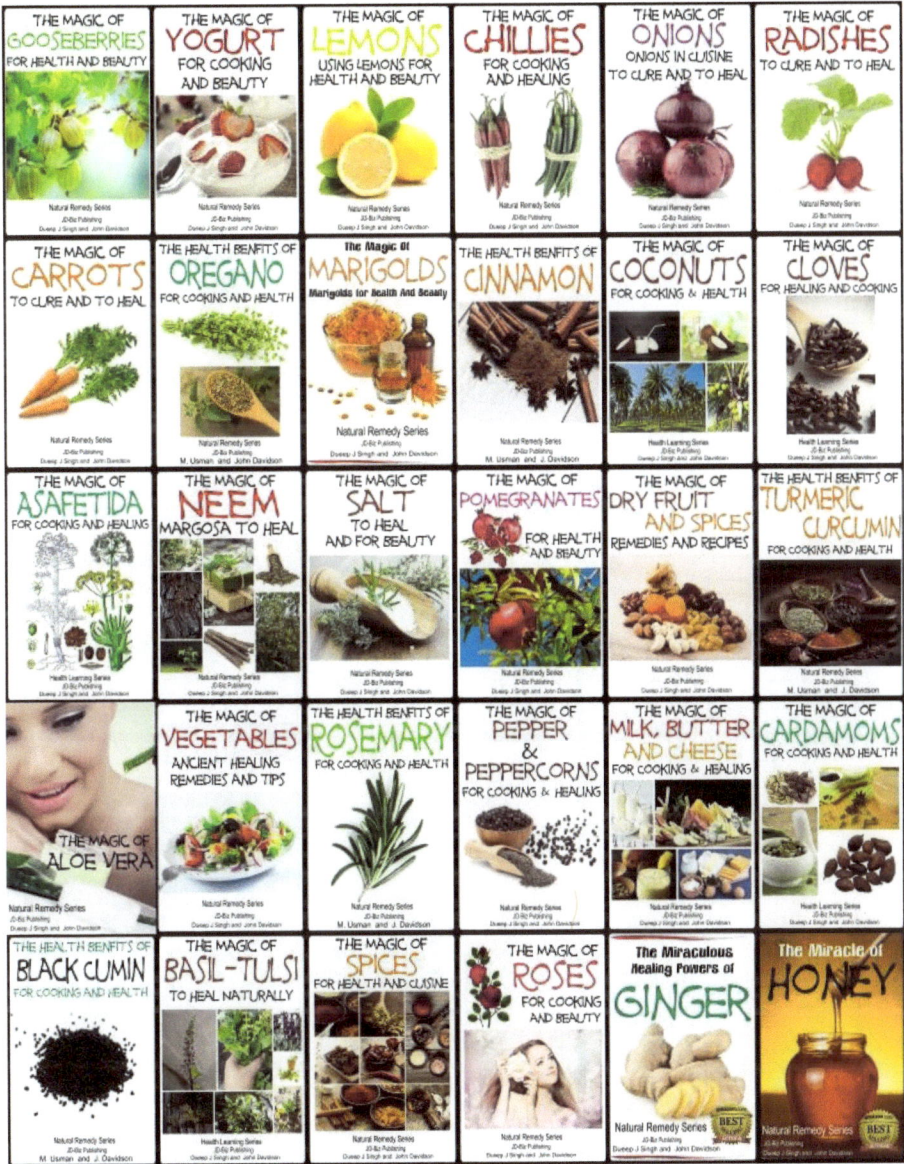

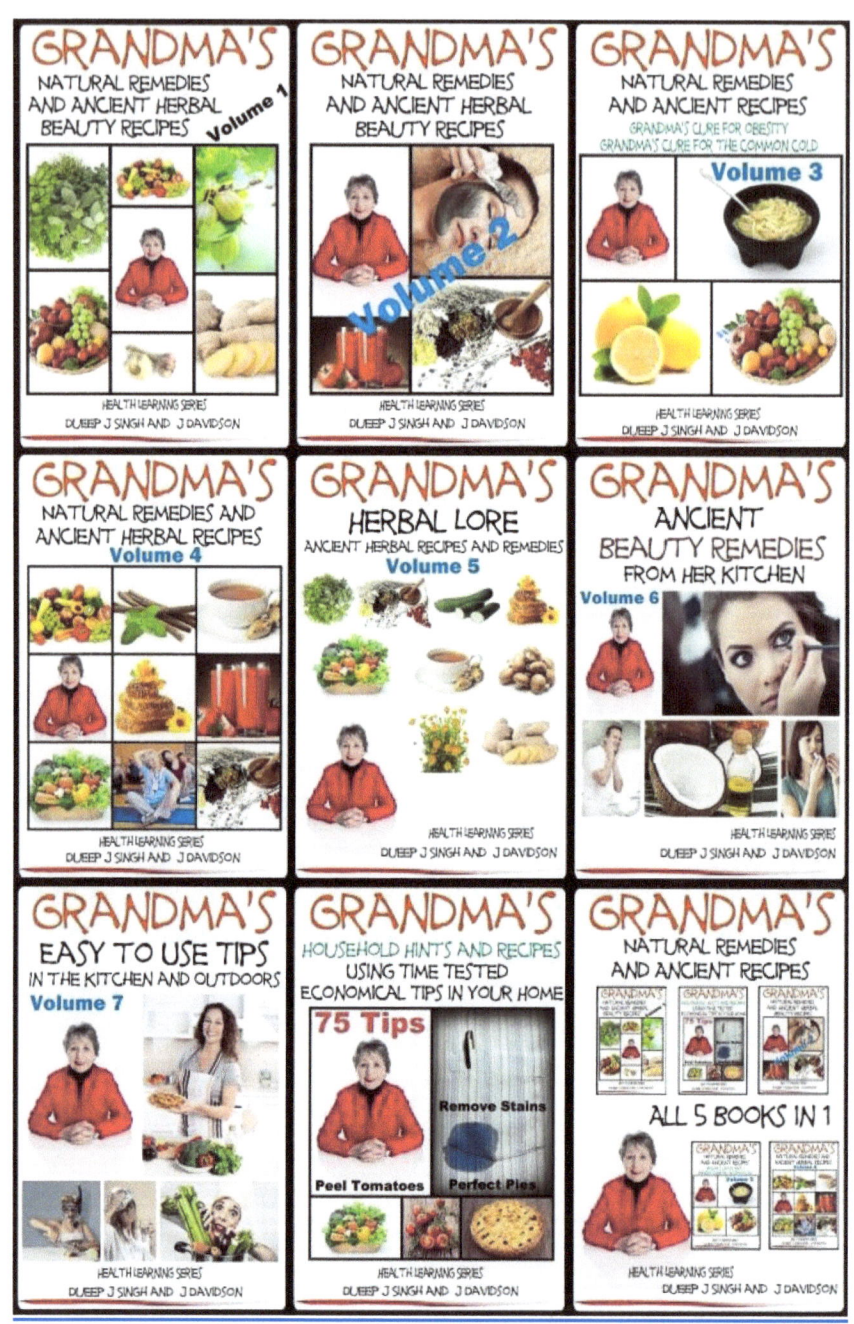

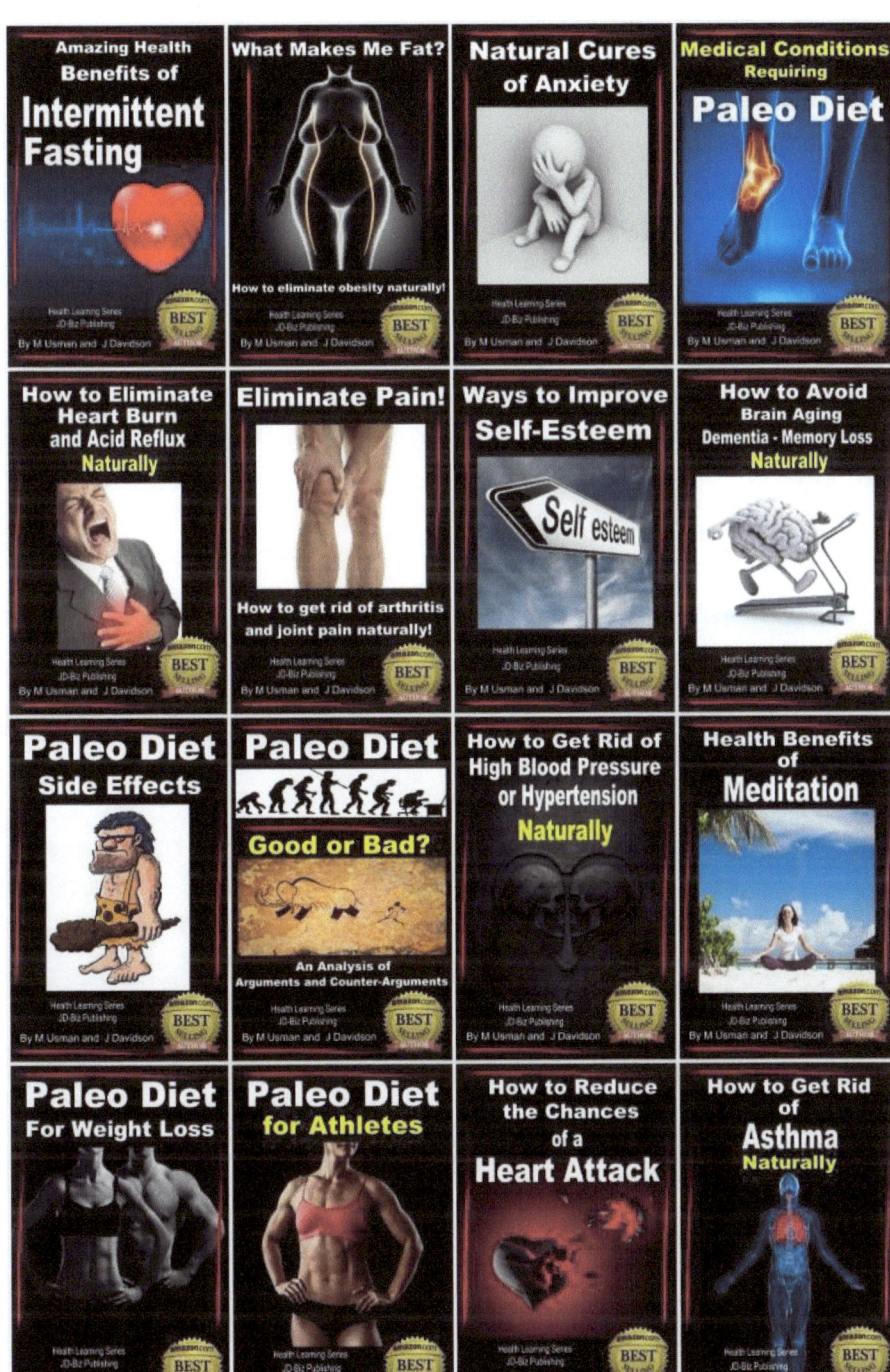

Amazing Animal Book Series

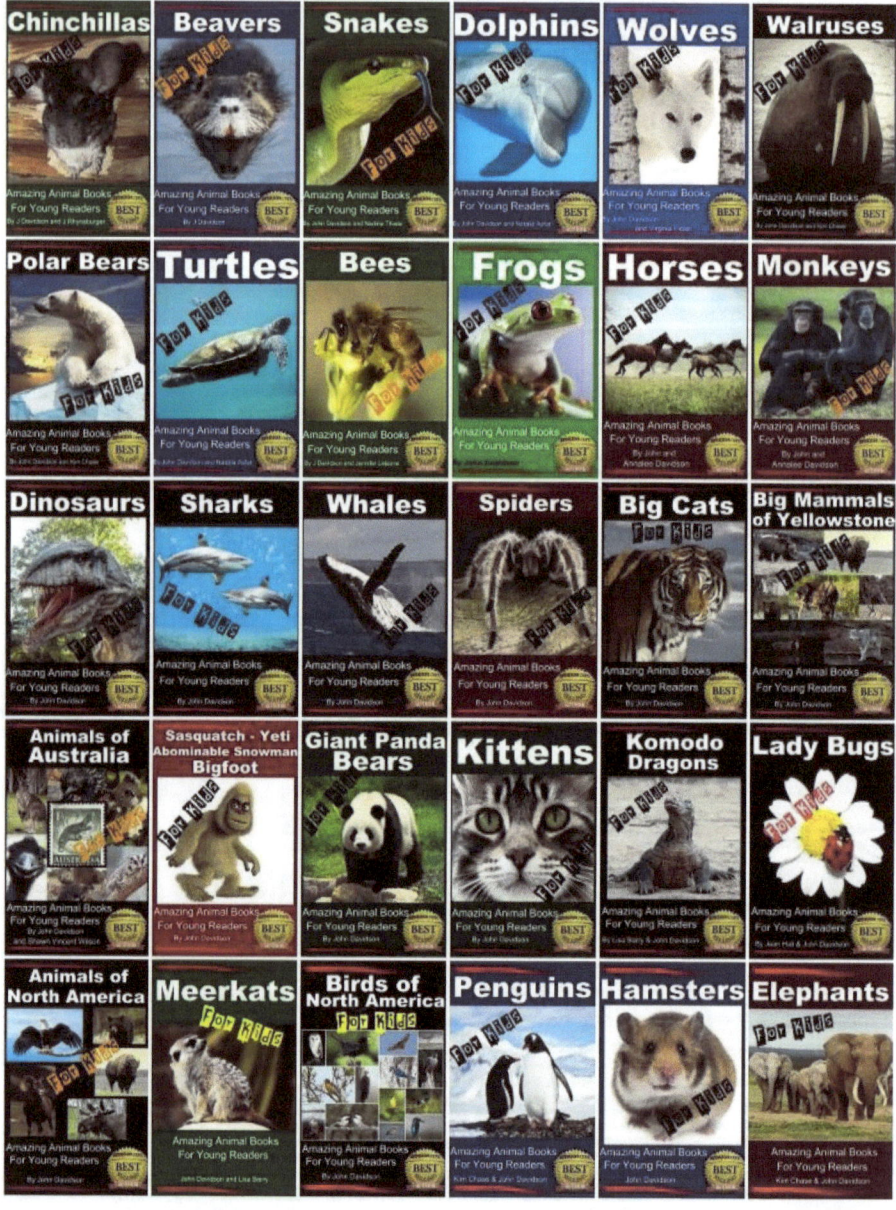

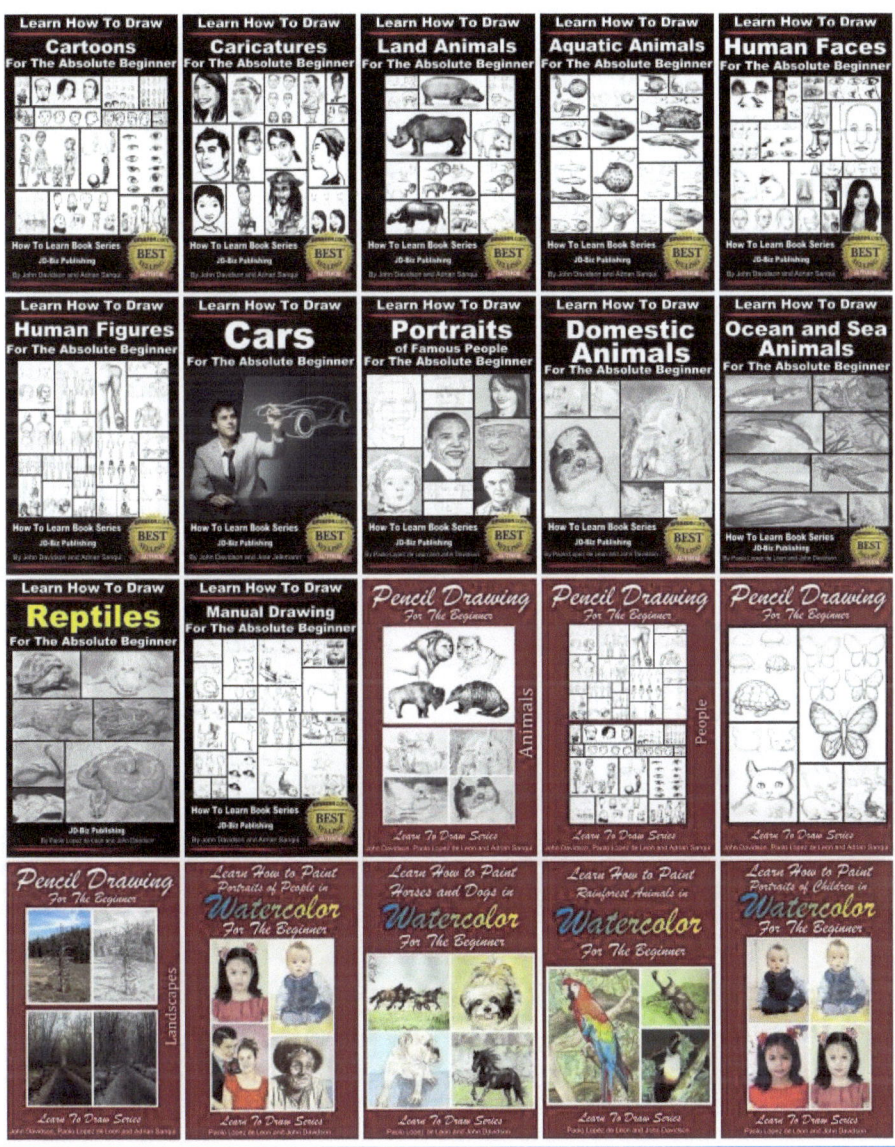

How to Build and Plan Books

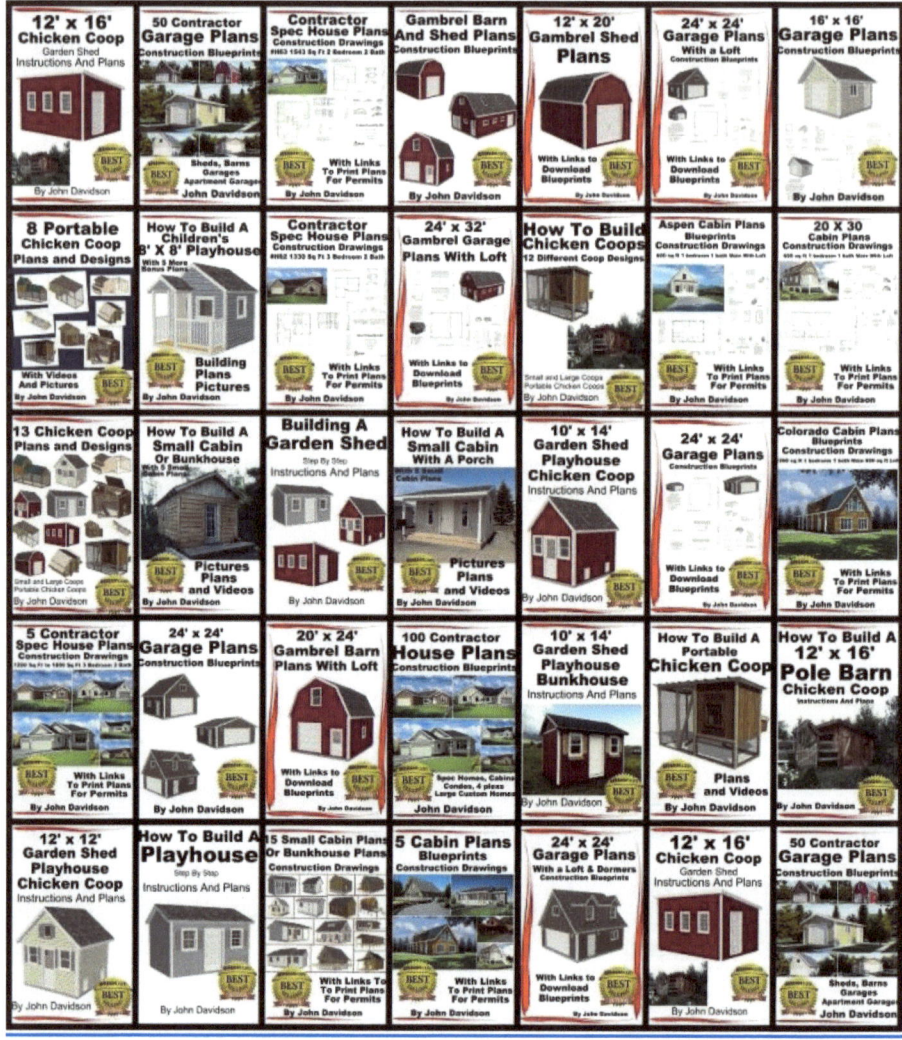

Entrepreneur Book Series

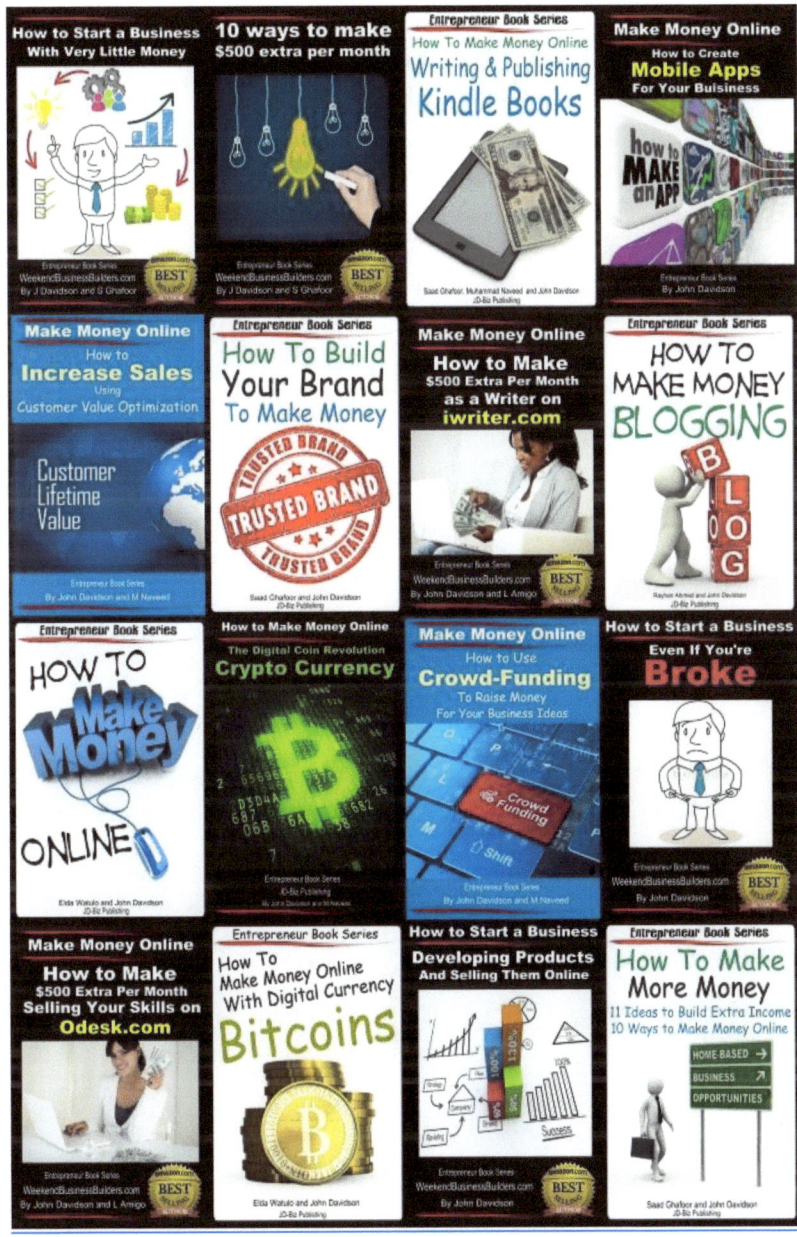

Our books are available at

1. Amazon.com

2. Barnes and Noble

3. Itunes

4. Kobo

5. Smashwords

6. Google Play Books

Download Free Books!

http://MendonCottageBooks.com

Publisher

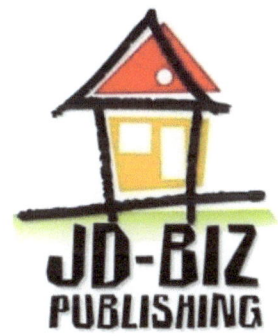

JD-Biz Corp

P O Box 374

Mendon, Utah 84325

http://www.jd-biz.com/

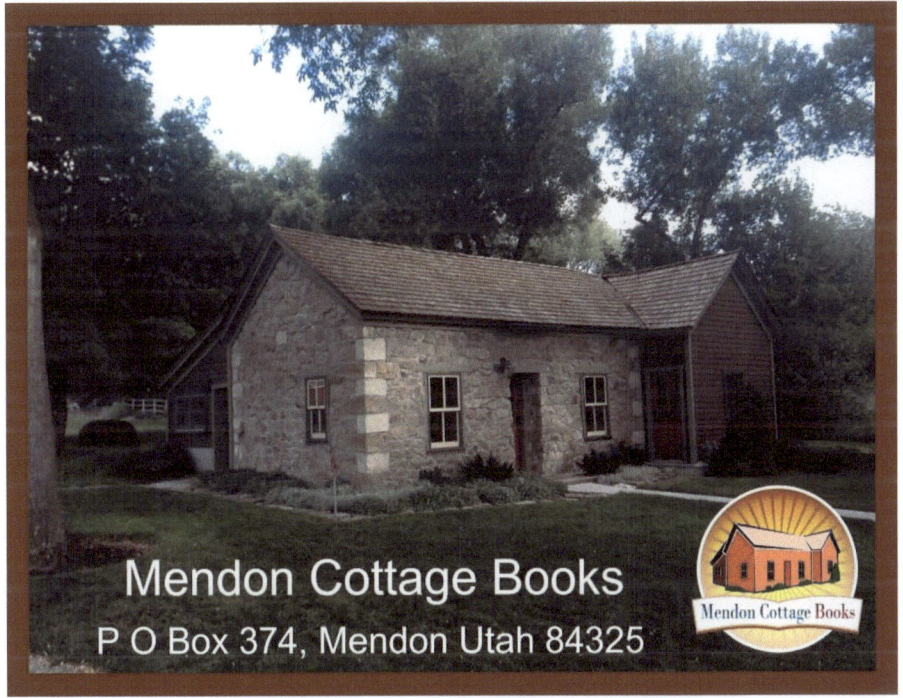